ART OF

SUPER-REALIZATION

INITIATION

By

SWAMI YOGANANDA

—✦—

This sacred lesson is meant only for the devoted Yogoda
student who would, untiringly and unceasingly,
seek God until he finds Him

—✦—

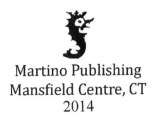

Martino Publishing
Mansfield Centre, CT
2014

Martino Publishing
P.O. Box 373,
Mansfield Centre, CT 06250 USA

ISBN 978-1-61427-734-7

© 2014 Martino Publishing

Cover design by T. Matarazzo

Printed in the United States of America On 100% Acid-Free Paper

ART OF

SUPER-REALIZATION

INITIATION

By

SWAMI YOGANANDA

—◆—

This sacred lesson is meant only for the devoted Yogoda
student who would, untiringly and unceasingly,
seek God until he finds Him

—◆—

Published By
YOGODA SAT-SANGA SOCIETY
3880 San Rafael Avenue
Mount Washington
Los Angeles, Calif.

ART OF SUPER-REALIZATION

By Swami Yogananda

INITIATION

Invocation

O Heavenly Father, Jesus, Prophet of my religion, Prophets of all religions, Supreme Master Babaji, Great Master Lahiri Mahasaya, Swami Sriyukteswar Giriji, and you, my Guru (Preceptor), free my spiritual path from all difficulties, and lead me to the shores of eternal wisdom and bliss.

Babaji

Babaji is the Supreme Master of the Yogoda Sat-Sanga movement in America and India. His disciples claim that he is living an extraordinarily long life. It was he who gave this lesson to Lahiri Mahasaya, who revived the art of Super-Realization and practical Yoga in a sweeping way in Bengal and India, teaching thousands of disciples.

Lahiri Mahasaya

Lahiri Mahasaya was an ideal prophet and a Christ-like man, while married and performing the duties of ordinary life. We can picture saints in the forests, but when we find them in the jungles of civilization we can hold hopes of spiritual salvation for the worldly man.

1

Swami Sriyukteswar

Disciple of Lahiri Mahasaya is Swami Sriyukteswar Giriji, my Master. The inspiration and command for the spread of Yogoda Sat-Sanga in America is due to Babaji and Swami Sriyukteswar Giriji. It was Swami Sriyukteswar Giriji who chose Swami Yogananda as the only representative to spread the message of lost Yoga and Super-Art of Salvation. Swami Sriyukteswar Giriji is one of the world's intellectual and spiritual giants. In him East and West meet. He came to unite the best in Eastern and Western civilizations. His message combines the necessary lessons on material and spiritual life, bridging the chasm existing between theology and true inner realization. Yogoda teachings emphasize the necessity of concentrating on the technique of salvation and not on unproved religious beliefs.

Sat-Sanga

Sat-Sanga is fellowship of religions and includes the good in all.

Yogoda

Yogoda is the scientific technique for developing body, mind and soul harmoniously. It is the method for recharging the body, mind and soul batteries from inner cosmic energy. It is the universal technique of salvation, the royal highway in which all theological bypaths conjoin.

Swami

Swami is a title received from another Swami, signifying the highest order of renunciation. Swami means master of himself, or one who is trying to master himself. A Swami recognizes no other family than the entire human family. Only a Swami can ordain another Swami.

Yogi

A Yogi is he who scientifically unites his soul with Spirit through the teachings of a Guru. A Yogi may be a worldly man or a man of renunciation.

Guru and Disciple Versus Teacher and Student

Guru means preceptor. One can have many teachers in the beginning of the study of difficult teachings, but one can have only one Guru, who leads him to God-consciousness. The Guru is the vehicle through which God redeems a disciple from mental bondage. He who receives this lesson ought to take the preceptor of this lesson as Guru. He would then be known as a Yogi or Yogodan or a Yogoda disciple. One can have many teachers before he settles down to one path and one Guru. Until he takes the one path and the one Guru, he is called a student, not a disciple.

Yogoda Student

A Yogoda student is a Yogi.

Student

One who receives the Yogoda lessons is only a student.

Disciple

A disciple is he who advances in the Yogoda faith and strictly follows the path of Super-Realization as given in this lesson and as directed by one Guru. One has to live a life of discrimination in order to be a Swami or a Yogi.

3

SUPER-REALIZATION

Posture and Preparation Necessary to the Correct Methods of Practicing the Exercises Given in This Lesson on the Great Art of Super-Realization

Preparation

1. Face east, sitting on a straight, armless chair, over which a woolen blanket has been placed, running down under the feet.

2. Take a teaspoonful of melted butter (unsalted) or olive oil. This is to grease the throat. The butter or oil should not be swallowed quickly. Sip it slowly. It is extremely important to observe this rule, as the throat must be well greased.

There should be no deviation from any of the methods given in this lesson. There are few rules. Obey them strictly.

Posture

3. Correct posture: Spine erect; shoulder blades together; palms upward, resting on thighs; chest out; abdomen in; chin parallel to the ground; relax whole body, keeping spine straight.

The correct posture is extremely important. It will be almost altogether ineffectual to perform this exercise with bent spine.

4. With spine erect, relax all muscles and limbs. During the practice of this lesson the spine often bends forward

4

unconsciously through bad habits. Straighten it as often as it bends, to gain the desired results.

After the correct posture has been attained, and all muscles and limbs are relaxed, practice the following exercise, called Kriya, for magnetizing the spine.

He who practices Kriya is a Kriyaban or a true Brahmin or true twice-born Christian, or a man of realization. He is born again as spoken of in the Christian Bible:

"Except ye be born again, ye cannot enter the kingdom of heaven."

The physical birth is given by the father, the spiritual birth is given by the Guru (preceptor), the one individual who is able to lead the disciple to God-consciousness. One may have had many teachers before, but when he finds his Guru he becomes the only one throughout life. The Guru is the vehicle of God through which God teaches and calls the disciple to Himself.

KRIYA CONSISTS OF THREE PARTS
Part 1—Kriya Proper

The first part of Kriya, or Kriya proper, teaches the method of mentally feeling the spine by passing or circulating life current lengthwise around it.

The purpose of Kriya is to magnetize the spine by circulating life current lengthwise around it, and thereby withdrawing the life current from the senses and involuntary organs and concentrating it in the spine. This also helps to change the center of consciousness from the body and senses to the spine.

5

The spinal column should be imagined as hollow when circulating the breath and life current lengthwise in and around it.

Method

1. With half-opened eyes fixed at the Will Center (the point between the eyebrows), concentrate on the whole spinal column, and imagine it to be a hollow tube running from the point between the eyebrows to the coccyx.

2. Inhale, feeling the breath pass through the inside of this imaginary hollow spinal canal, with the sound of "Hau" (made by the expanded throat), thinking and feeling a cool breath and current starting from the coccyx at the terminal of the spine and moving upward until it reaches the top of the tube imagined as running up to the point between the eyebrows. The duration of inhalation, with the thought of pulling the breath and current upward, must be ten to fifteen counts.

When the current and breath have reached the top of the spinal tube, the point between the eyebrows, slowly exhale, sending the breath and current over the forehead, through the cerebrum and on down the back of the spinal column to the coccyx. While exhaling, the current and breath must be felt as a fine, thread-like, tepid (slightly warm) stream slowly going over the spine downward to the coccyx. As you exhale, imagining the current to flow downward over the back of the spine, make the sound of "E" with the breath.

When you inhale and exhale continuously, you quickly convert the oxygen into life force, especially recharging

6

lungs and blood. Focusing the vision and the will at the point between the eyebrows, and imagining the circulation of the current and breath in and around the spine, will create a positive and a negative pole and bring about the actual circulation of this current.

The Will Center becomes the positive pole and the coccygeal plexus becomes the negative pole. The current thus created becomes a magnet of energy which draws more energy from the nervous system and from the Cosmic Source. By this method the adept is enabled to project this energy from the medulla into Cosmic Energy. It is then that this energy in the body loses its limitations and becomes identified with Cosmic Energy. This is what is meant by Pranayama or control of life force in spine and heart and nervous system, which results in breathlessness and the calming down of heart and lungs. It is then that the life force, which is dependent on oxygen, loses its breath-slavery and moves spiritward.[1]

While inhaling and exhaling, imagine that the breath during inhalation is going upward from the coccyx to the point between the eyebrows; and during exhalation, imagine that it is moving downward over the back of the spinal column. The breath actually does not circulate around the whole length of the spine, but the increased life force derived from the transmuted breath is directed by will and

[1] Many think that control of life force means control of breath. That is wrong. The real meaning of Pranayama, according to Patanjali, the founder of Yoga philosophy, is the gradual cessation of breathing, the discontinuance of inhalation and exhalation. Trying to control the life force by holding the breath in the lungs is extremely unscientific.

7

visualization to circulate lengthwise, within and without, through the inner and over the outer side of the spinal cord continuously during Kriya. This converts the entire spine into a magnet which draws all the bodily current away from the senses and nerves. The five telephones of the senses—touch, taste, smell, hearing and sight—are thus disconnected and the attention freed from the invasion of the senses. This is also the greatest psycho-physical method for actually reversing the searchlights of life forces, consciousness and the senses from matter to spirit.

Drawing up and feeling a cool current and the breath within the inside of the spine, feeling a cool current from the coccyx to the point between the eyebrows, and spraying the current and breath as tepid over the back of the spinal tube from the point between the eyebrows down to the coccyx, is equal to one complete Kriya exercise. This exercise should be performed from one to fourteen times in immediate succession, morning and evening.

Remember, there are two indications of the correct practice of Kriya.

1. During inhalation, the upward-floating breath and current should produce a cool sensation throughout the entire length of the imaginary hollow in the spinal column, from the coccyx to the point between the eyebrows. (The inhalation must be accompanied throughout by the deep sound of "Hau" made by the expanded throat.)

2. During exhalation, the downward-floating breath and current should be felt as a tepid, fine, thread-like sensation, accompanied by the sound of "E" (made by the

8

expanded throat). Do not jerk the chest by moving it up and down with inhalation and exhalation, while practicing Kriya.

3. Always keep the throat expanded, during this exercise. The expansion should be like that experienced in rolling the tongue backward toward the uvula. You may practice Kriya with an expanded throat by rolling the tongue backward.

4. Drawing the breath and current upward must be accompanied by a deep, full sound of "Hau," made by the throat. Likewise, in sending the current downward over the spinal column, it must be fine, thread-like and tepid. This exhalation must be accompanied by the sound of "E," made by the throat.

The repetition of Kriya twelve to fourteen times equals one year's natural evolution in development of body, mind and soul. The life current quickly spiritualizes the spine and brain, which in turn spiritualize the whole body. Hindu Yogis state that this current actually changes the atomic composition of the body cells.

Ordinarily the progress of the human body, mind and soul keeps pace with the revolutions of the earth around the sun. (Of course, this natural progress is retarded if disease, accidents, despondency or ignorance be permitted to invade the body, mind or soul.) Just as the earth's complete revolution around the sun produces one year's effects in the human body, so the Yogis discovered that the time of human evolution could be quickened greatly by revolving the life-force (the earthly physical energy) around the elliptical path of the spinal cord and its six centers, upward from the coccyx to the point between the eyebrows, and downward from the point between the eyebrows to the coccyx, with the soul as the central sun.

The solar year through outside influences of rays and vibrations quickens the body, mind and soul to a certain state in a year's time. The Yogis found that the same result of one year's complete bodily evolution and spiritual change can be brought about by internal methods for energizing and spiritualizing the spine which is extremely sensitive. This quickening of evolution can be accomplished only if Kriya is practiced correctly, if the body is kept free from diseases and accidents, and the mind from disbelief and error.

Normally, the human body, brain, mind and soul undergo a complete change once every eight years, if the individual be progressive. The Scriptures say it requires about a million uninterrupted mundane years of human progressive natural evolution to clarify and sensitize and enlarge the brain, mind and soul capacity so that they can hold and reflect all the knowledge in the Universe. Ordinarily, the human brain is too limited even to hold all the words of an enlarged Webster Dictionary. Imagine what a highly developed brain is necessary to hold and express all knowledge. However, if Luther Burbank could bring a walnut tree to the fruit-bearing stage in five years instead of the normal ten to fifteen years, it is reasonable to suppose that there must be a scientific method for developing an all-wisdom-producing brain within a few years, instead of a million terrestrial years as usually required.

This is why the Yogis of India have devised this ingenious Kriya exercise for internally refining the brain and spine. Kriya is mathematical in its result. All who practice it correctly and regularly will learn this for themselves. By practicing Kriya correctly fourteen times, morning and evening, while in good health, the spine, brain and mind become completely changed. To bring about an equivalent change through natural evolution requires one year. Consequently, by practicing Kriya fourteen times in the morning and fourteen times in the evening, two years of natural evolution can be achieved in one day.

One must remember that one million years of evolution can be achieved in less than fifty years by perfecting one's technique, deepening concentration, and by increasing the number of times in the practice of Kriya. (This is not to be attempted without the permission of the Guru, which may be obtained after several months of faithful practice, by reporting on the state of your health and mind.)

You can also practice the lesson on the Art of Super-Realization, especially the Kriya, in the following way:

Sit upright. Expand your throat by rolling the tongue backward, keeping the mouth almost closed, and circulate the cool and tepid currents as directed to do in the other method of Kriya practice. While drawing the cool current upward from the coccyx to the medulla by the sound of "Hau," you can mentally chant Aum (Om) at each of the six centers. During exhalation, accompanied by the sound of "E," mentally chant Aum (Om) at each center as the tepid current flows downward. See following illustrations.

11

Kriya Proper

Expanded Throat

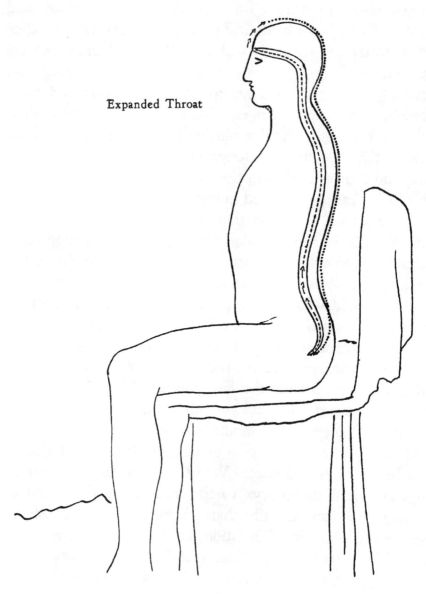

12

MAHA MUDRA EXERCISE

Part 2—Maha Mudra

This exercise is called Maha Mudra, or body-electri-fication and spine-straightening method.

Maha Mudra should be practiced on the floor on a woolen blanket.

The purpose of this exercise is to loosen the vertebræ and distribute the obstructed life current into the organs. Maha Mudra is performed in three parts, as follows:

(a)[1] Bend the left leg and sit on the sole of left foot. Bend the right knee upward, having right foot flat on the floor; place hands with fingers interlocked over right knee. Keep the spine straight. Inhale, cooling the inside of the cerebro-spinal tube as in Kriya, bringing the current up inside the tube to the forehead, between the eyebrows. Then, hold-ing the breath, bend head forward and downward, resting chin on chest, and stretch right leg forward, straight on floor. With both hands take hold of the great toe of the right foot, and pull it toward you. Count from one to six in this bent posture (breath still being held),[2] then sit up, straightening spine, and lifting the right knee upward (knee flexed) in comfortable position. Then exhale with the sound of "E" as in Kriya, sending the warm current over the out-side of the tube downward to the coccyx.[3]

(b) Repeat this same exercise by bending the right leg and foot and sitting on the sole of the right foot.

(c) Sit erect, both knees up, feet on the ground over a blanket. With fingers interlocked and placed over knees, draw current upward to the sound of "Hau" as in Kriya. Hold breath, bend head down, with chin on chest, then stretch both legs straight forward on the floor, keeping them together. Shift interlocked fingers to toes of both feet and, holding toes, pull them toward you.[1] Count from one to six, holding breath,[2] then sit up, straightening spine, and exhale with the sound of "E."[3]

Maha Mudra

EXERCISE (a)

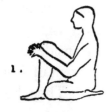 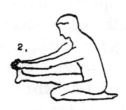 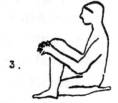

EXERCISE (b)

Same as exercise "a" but reversing leg positions.

EXERCISE (c)

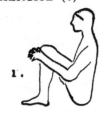 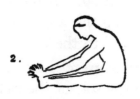 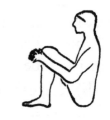

YOTI MUDRA

Part 3—Yoti Mudra

The purpose of the third part of Kriya is seeing the light by your own effort, or finding guidance through the spiritual eye.

1. Sit erect.

2. Put thumbs of both hands loosely over tragus of both ears.

3. Place first fingers lightly over the outer corners of the lids with gentle pressure.

4. Place middle fingers lightly over nostrils.

5. The position of third fingers should be over corners of the upper lip and that of the little fingers over the corners of the lower lip. With all fingers lightly held in these positions, inhale with the sound of "Hau," drawing current up through the cerebrospinal tube from the coccyx to the point between the eyebrows.

6. Hold breath.

7. Knit eyebrows tightly and quickly.

8. Press eyeballs gently, so they do not revolve or rotate.

9. Press all fingers firmly, closing mouth, nostrils, ears and eyes. Count from one to twelve or twenty-five, holding breath, and see the revolving light of the spiritual eye (the star of wisdom, the third eye, the dove descending from heaven, the single eye, the star of the East through which your wisdom must pass to meet Christ-Consciousness). The astral eye in the beginning will reveal astral lights. Then, by deeper concentration, this eye will become

spiritualized, revealing spirit. Watch the spiritual Aurora Borealis, then loosen fingers, while keeping them in the same position, and exhale, sending the current down over the spinal column with the sound of "E."

Repeat this exercise two or three times. Practice once just before going to bed.

Yoti Mudra

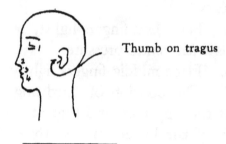

Thumb on tragus

KRIYA

General Remarks

By the correct practice of Kriya fourteen times, Maha Mudra twice, and Yoti Mudra twice, twelve years of evolution of body, mind and soul will be gained in a few minutes. Mind can do everything. Through this practice, the time limitation in evolution is overcome, and the receptive power of the spine, brain and mind is increased, so that the Yogi knows, sees and feels all from within. Yoga is the super-method by which the evolution of body, mind and soul can be quickened. That is how the attainment of wisdom and realization, which usually takes a million years and numerous incarnations of natural evolution, is possible in one lifetime.

By this exercise, the consciousness which is in the body, and which is identified with the senses, is transferred to the spine and the brain, and thus transmitted into Super-consciousness and Cosmic Consciousness.

Kriya is an initiation into Cosmic Consciousness, or the transfer of consciousness from the body to the spirit. In order to do this, one must transfer consciousness from the senses to the spine.

After practicing Kriya and resting for a short while, one is able to do inspired work in connection with literature, art or science. Then intuition develops of itself, without effort, because one's consciousness is transferred from the senses to the spine and brain.

Realization can come only by the development of one's intuition.

Remember that through the practice of this lesson you will contact Christ, and the prophets of this world, and through them you will find your union with God the Infinite Spirit.

While practicing Kriya feel the inspiration of God in the spine.

KRIYA

Practical Advice

1. Avoid excitement.
2. Do not lead unbalanced lives.
3. Observe strict moderation in everything, especially in sex life.

4. Do not practice Kriya during physical illness or while pain is felt in any part of the chest or body. Kriya presupposes sound health. However, do not seek excuses, but when able to do so, practice Kriya.

5. Kriya is meant to accelerate the forces of the body when in perfect health. Do not practice this exercise when suffering from colds, throat troubles, bronchitis, tuberculosis, or any other ailment of the throat, lungs or alimentary canal. (The exercises given in the first Yogoda Course are for restoring and maintaining the body in perfect health.)

This method teaches that human consciousness is usually located and attached to the spinal vertebræ in the body. Therefore, the soul forgets its Omnipresent Kingdom and becomes identified with the small surface of the body.

This Kriya method of magnetizing spinal column teaches one to transfer consciousness from sense and body centers to the spinal and brain centers, through which the Spirit descends into the body.

CPSIA information can be obtained
at www.ICGtesting.com
Printed in the USA
LVHW100102080123
736644LV00001B/88